Essential Oils for Diffusers
40 Amazing Blends and Recipes

Table of Contents

Introduction

Essential oils are natural oils that are typically obtained through some processes such as distillation, from plants. Essential oils do have some characteristic odour of plant or any other source from which they are extracted from. Essential oils have been used for thousands of years in the cure of several ailments, and were heavily relied upon for spiritual and emotional uplifting.

Scientifically, an essential oil can be defined as a concentrated hydrophobic liquid that contains the aromatic compounds from the plant source. They are often regarded as volatile oils or ethereal oils, depending on the plant from which they are obtained. They are the main fragrant that contains the highly concentrated constituents of their plant sources.

Essential oils play several biological roles in plants; they do help plants attract insect pollinators, through the aroma they produce. They also give some flowers, their characteristic unique bright colours. A single component of an essential oil can attract millions of pollinating insects to a plant.

Essential oils can also serve as the defense protector of a plant. The terpenoid compounds in plants are capable of repelling insects , birds or other predators of plants. The anti-fungal and anti-bacterial natures of essential oils make them the only reliable natural defense mechanisms for plants.

In the modern world, essential oils are more important than mere medicinal or rejuvenating compounds, their wonderful and fascinating aroma , make it possible for cosmetic companies to rely on them for perfumes, fragrances and makeups. Essential oils are normally available all through the parts of the plant but they are mostly concentrated in the leaves, stems and flowers.

One of the importance of diffusing your essential oils is that it helps you create a perfect balance and mix of two similar or different essential oils, therefore you can maximize the benefits in one if the benefit is not found in the other essential oil within the diffusion.

Secondly, diffusing essential oil can save you the time of diffusing too much of slowly extracting oils. If you use steam or water distillation for instance, you will notice that the speed of extraction of oils are different, but diffusion will help you extract substantial amount of one oil without waiting for the whole day to extract everything, knowing fully well that you can mix them.

Essential oil have remained the oldest and most trusted therapeutic treatment substances from ages, therefore you can rely on them to deliver, especially when you stick to the recommended doses highlighted in this piece of book.

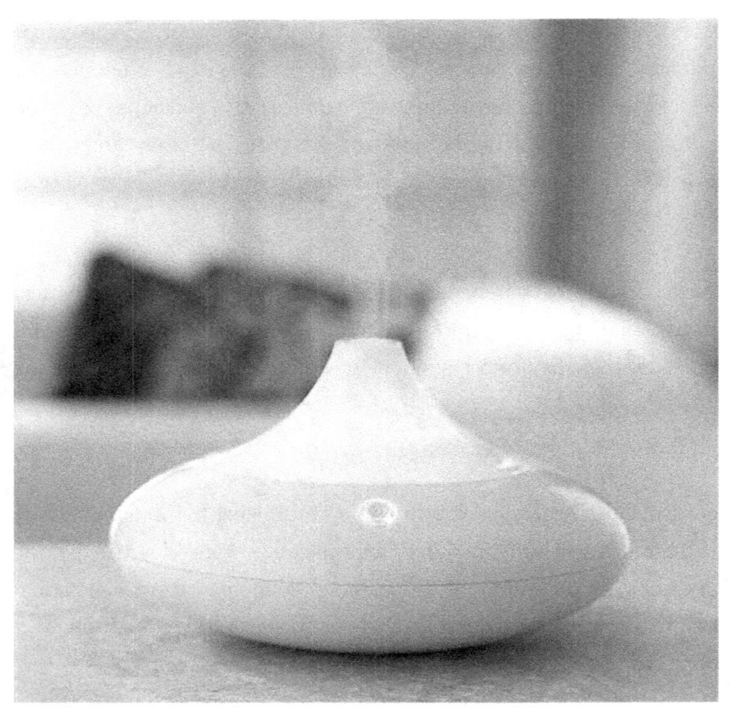

Chapter 1 Importance of diffused essential oils for healthy living

The diffusion of essential oil comes with numerous benefits, first it helps you reduce the risks attached to the volatility of the compounds of the essential oils , thus you can store the oils safely. You can also diffuse essential oil to increase its power of de-odourization and healing effects. If you have some allergy reactions, such as wheezing, then you may have to diffuse your oils to provide instant relief against such allergies.

In order to promote a calm and stress-free environment around your home, you need to diffuse essential oils. For instance, essential oils of plants such as Chamomile Lemon, Lavender, and Patchouli , can help produce a calming and stress-free environment. As a matter of fact, the diffusion of these essential oils will definitely make your house members and friends smell fresh and clean when they leave the place.

To enjoy the best uplifting therapy, make sure you go for essential oils such as Citrus fresh, Frankincense, Lemon and Bergamot oils. To boost your creativity levels, you should go for Bergamot and Jasmine essential oils- inhaling the scent of these essential oils can increase the speed of your thinking immediately.

One of the main importance of diffusing essential oil is that it helps you get all the benefits of the essential oils. When you get an essential oil from the store, you should not release it into your home directly because you may release some harmful chemicals at high concentrations, but with a diffuser, you can reduce the concentration of the oils by mixing it with other oils.

For relaxing, some of the essential oils you should consider for diffusion are; Lavender, Clary sage and Geranium. Diffusing your essential oil is quite simple, and the most important step is to add the essential oils into the diffuser, starting with the most volatile.

The diffuser works by simply pushing the essential oil into the air, before dispersing them across a space . Take note that the effectiveness of you diffuser to diffuse essential oil will depend on the distance and length of time the diffuser use to dispense its content.

It is important that you consider different diffuser and the environment for which you will use it. For larger spaces, cold-water diffuser may be the best option. There are basically two rules you must follow in diffusing essential oils;

1. You must use only therapeutic grade essential oils only, and
2. You must not heat the essential oil because you want to disperse its fragrance.

Diffusing essential oil is definitely the best possible way of drawing out all the benefits in such oils.

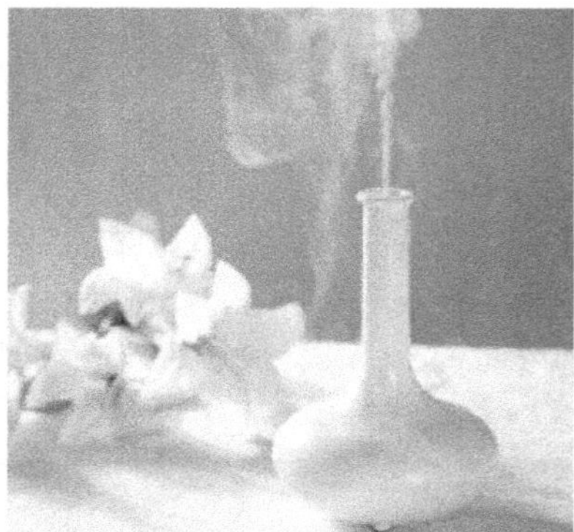

Chapter 2 Diffused essential oil recipes for treating stress, common diseases and infection

The procedure for diffusing essential oils is very simple, you need to get a diffuser , then measure your essential oils that you want to diffuse and add them in the diffuser . The diffuser has a handle that pushes the essential oils into the air and disperse them across the space. You need to set your diffuser in such a way that you can regulate the distance and length of time by which the essential oils are released.

Recipe #1: The Calming diffuser blend

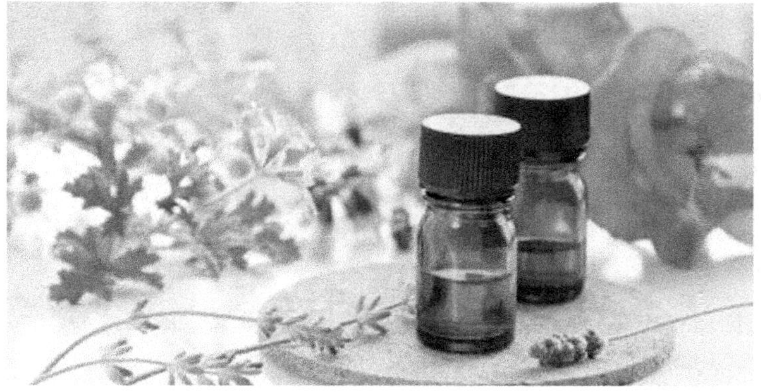

This is a blend of essential oils for relieving stress, and anxiety.

Ingredients:

- 4 drops of Roman Chamomile,
- 2 drops of Clary Sage,
- 3 drops of lavender,
- 2 drops of, and
- 1 drop of Ylang ylang.

Peppermint Essential Oil Uses

Curb Appetite

Headaches / Migraines

Cough / Congestion

Nausea / Motion Sickness

Refresh / Invigorate

Concentration / Focus

This recipe is perfect for strengthening respiratory functioning especially during the flu and cold seasons.

Ingredients:

- 1 drop of lime,
- 1 drop of lemon oil,
- 2 drops of,
- 1 drop of Rosemary essential oil, and
- 1 drop of Eucalyptus essential oil.

Recipe #3: The Cold and Flu combating essential oil recipe

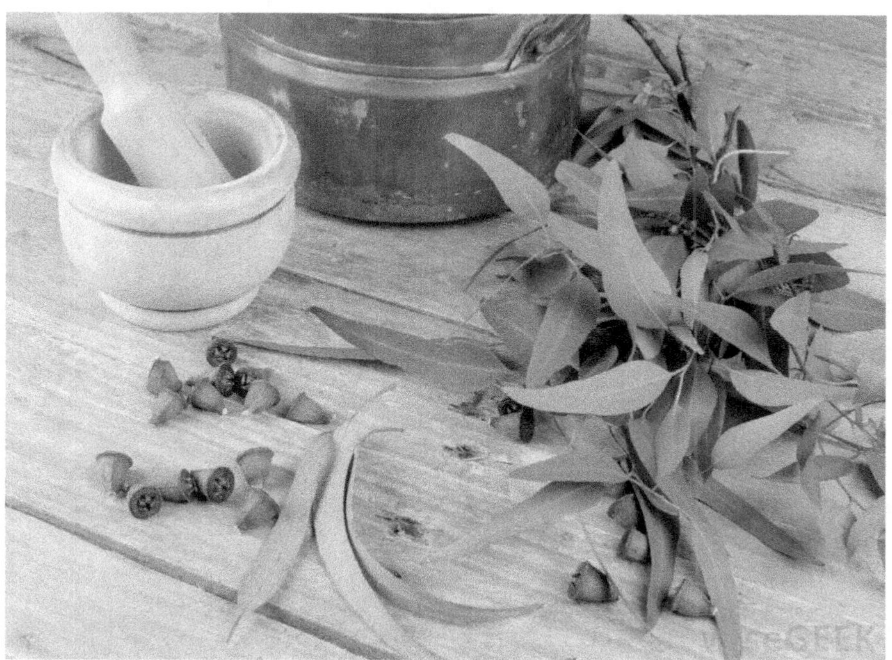

Speed up your recovery against cold and flu, you should have a blend of these essential oils in your diffuser;

Ingredients:

- 5 drops of lavender,
- 3 drops of Ravensara essential oil,
- 5 drops of Eucalyptus essential oil,
- 2 drops of Bay Laurel essential oils.

Recipe #4: Symptoms of allergies relief essential oil blend

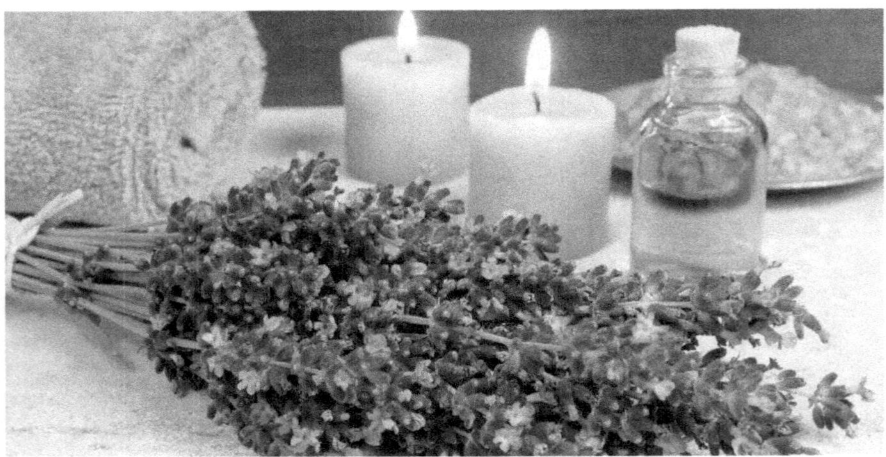

This perfect blend of essential oil can help ease off symptoms of allergic reactions

Ingredients

- 2 drops of peppermint oil,
- 2 drops of, and
- 2 drops of lemon essential oils.

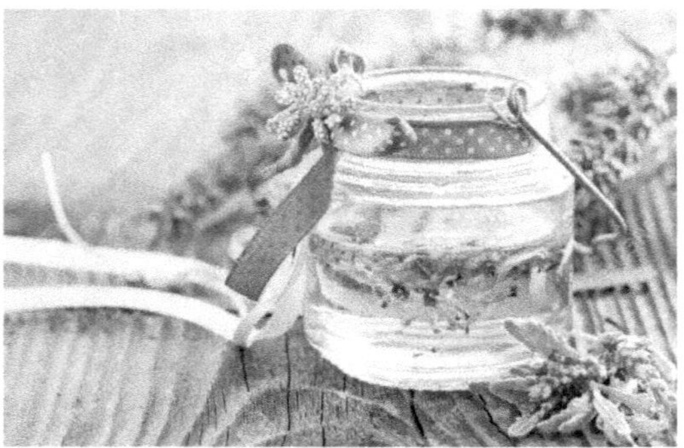

Recipe #5: Sleep apnea treatment essential oil recipe

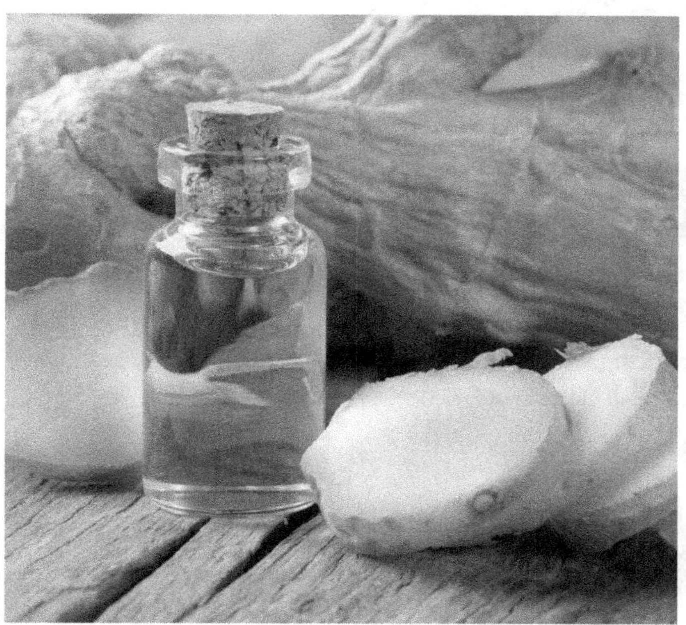

If you have problems getting good quality sleep, you can blend these basic relaxing and metal health stimulating essential oils in your diffuser;

Ingredients:

- 2 drop of marjoram oil,
- 2 drops of orange oil,
- 2 drops of Lavender oil,
- 2 drops of Bergamot oil,
- 2 drops of lime oil,
- 2 drops of grapefruit oil, and
- 2 drops of Ginger oil.

Recipe #6: Anti-bacteria formulation recipe

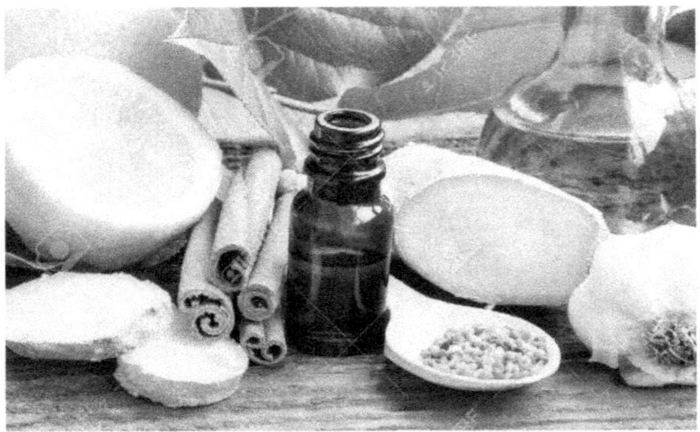

Essential oils do have anti-microbial qualities that can be as potent as some synthetic antibiotics, in the treatment of bacterial infection.

Ingredients:

- 6 drops of grapefruit oil
- 4 drops of Ginger root oil,
- 4 drops of lime essential oil,
- 4 drops of.

Recipe # 7: Muscle spasms, stomach upset and digestive problems

There are some powerful essential oils that can help provide relief against tensions in the muscles, nervous system and some organs. The combination effect of these essential oils will provide a lasting effect that can be cherished for a long time.

Ingredients:

- 2 drops of lavender,
- 2 drops of Cedarwood, and
- 2 drops of Marjoram.

Recipe #8: sore throat and respiratory problems

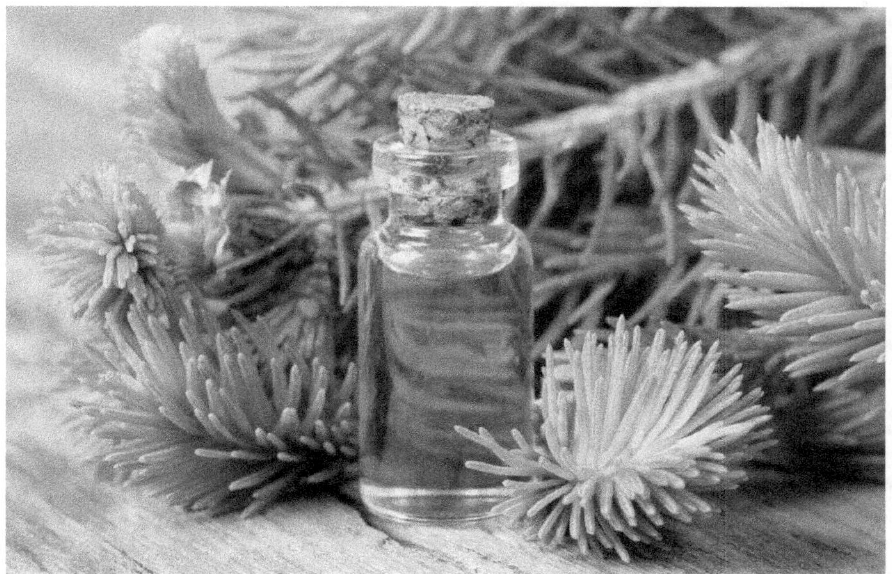

We all know that the combine power of lemon and Ginger can help provide soothing relief against respiratory disorders such as sore throat and flu symptoms. The addition of other ingredients such as Cyprus and White fir will provide extra energy for your body and mind.

Ingredients:

- 1 drop of white fir essential oil,
- 2 drops of lemon essential oil,
- 1 drop of ginger essential oil,
- 1 drop of, and
- 1 drop of Cyprus essential oil.

Chapter 3 Diffused essential oil recipes for skin and hair treatments

Hair losses and skin problems such as age spots, premature wrinkles and dry skin are just few of the common problems that can be treated with the use of essential oils. Some of the best recipes for these ailments include the following;

Recipe #9: Skin softening and healing recipe

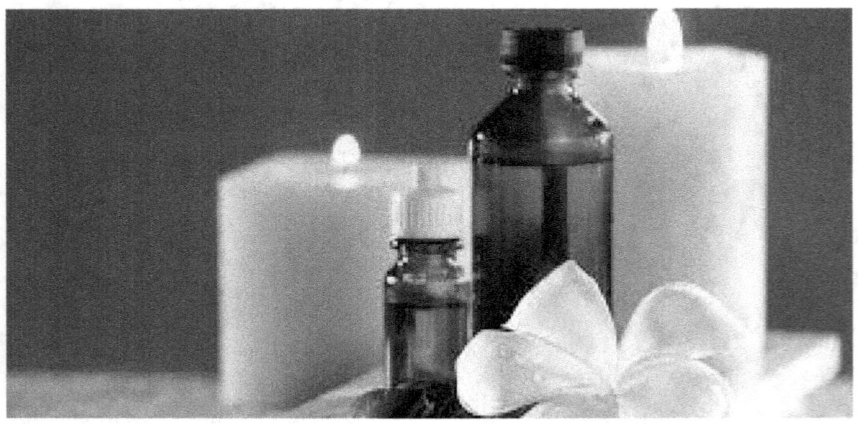

Dilute these essential oil mixes into your bath and enjoy the aromatherapy power of skin rejuvenating essential oils.

Ingredient:

- 8-10 drops of lavender essential oil,
- 2-3 drops of Palmarosa oil,
- 2-3 drops of Rose Geranium essential oils.

Recipe #10: The skin dullness treatment (for dry skins)

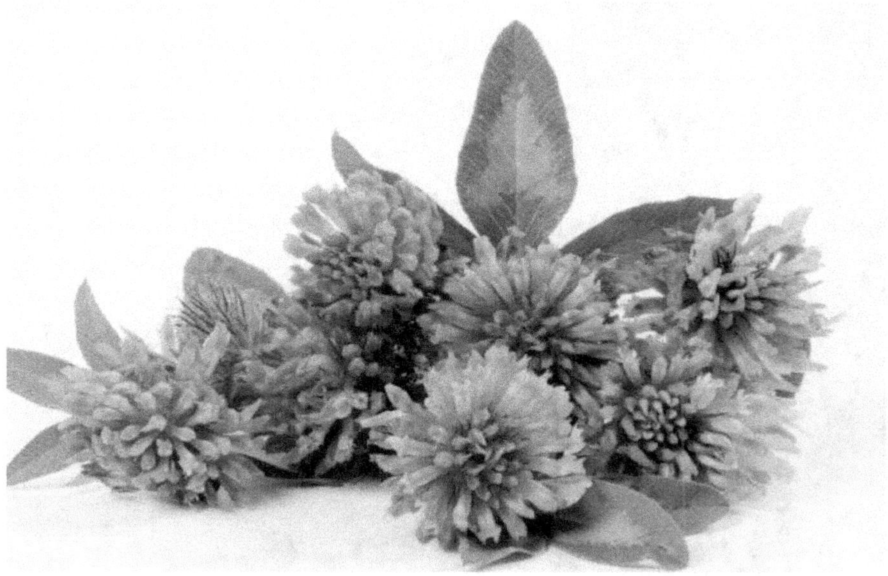

A mix of clove with Cinnamon and orange can help rejuvenate a dry skin and make it supple within few minutes. Clove contains powerful antioxidants that destroy oxidative stress on the skin, while the wild orange helps purify skin pores.

Ingredients:

- 2 drops of wild orange,
- 2 drops of Cinnamon, and
- 2 drops of oil extracts of Clove.

Recipe #11: The hair regrowth formula

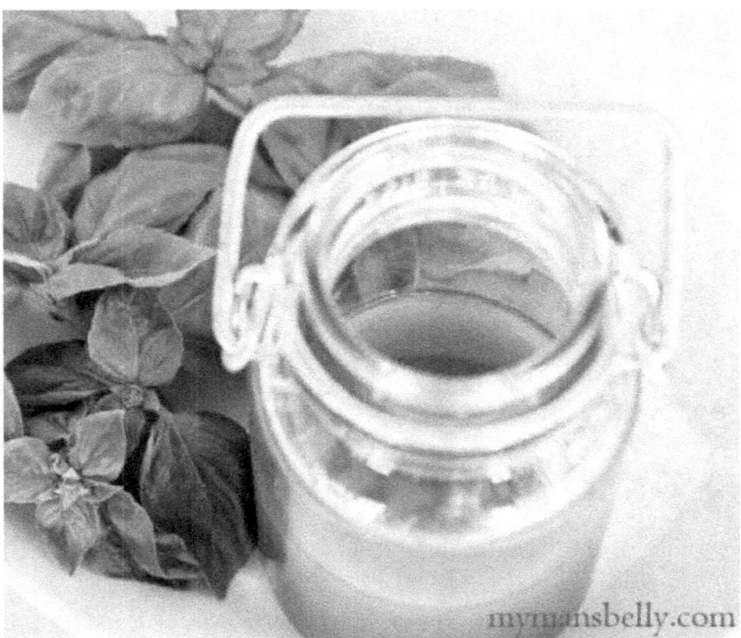

One essential ingredient you will find in most hair treatment products nowadays is the Basil, which is good for oily hair and also promote hair growth by stimulating circulation.

Ingredients:

- 4 drops of,
- 2 drops of Chamomile.

Recipe #12: Perfect essential oil for dandruffs and other hair problems

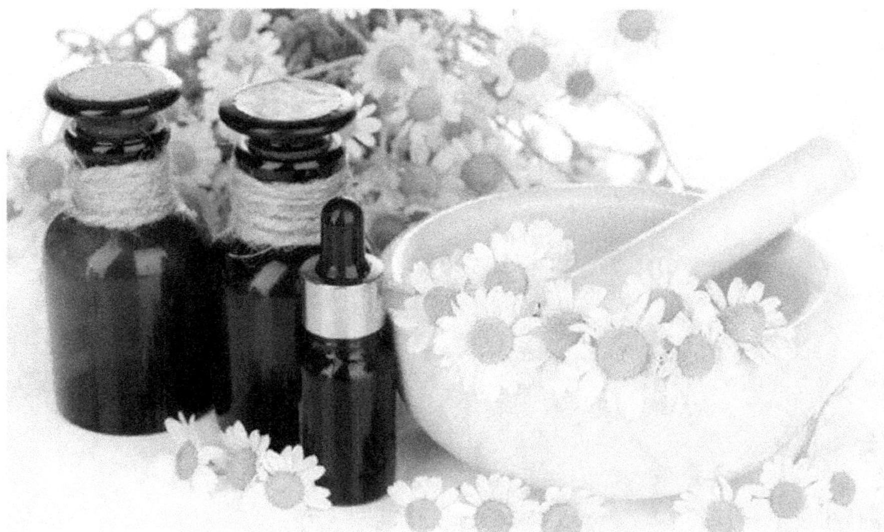

Do feel like you have a sore on your scalp or you are losing hair due to stubborn dandruffs? Clinical researches has shown that essential oils extracted from potent plants such as Chamomile, Clary sage and Cedarwood, can help clear off issues on the scalp and within hair strands.

Ingredients:

- 3 drops of cedarwood oil,
- 3 drops of Clary sage essential oil,
- 2 drops of Chamomile essential oil, and
- 2 drops of Eucalyptus.

Recipe #13: The perfect recipe for oily hair

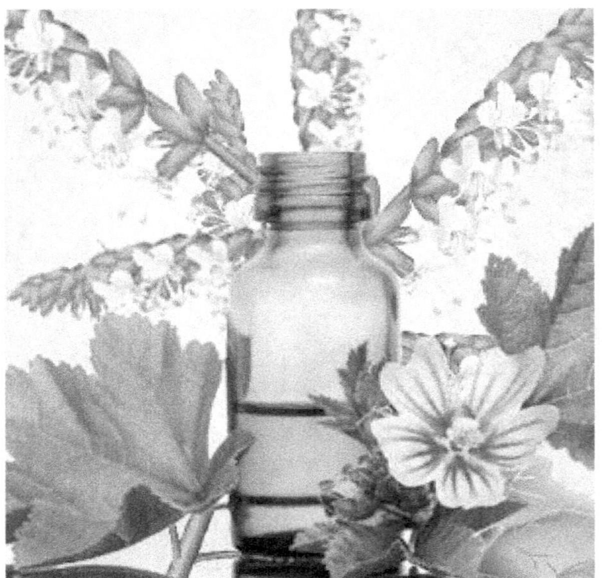

Oily hair is always messy, as dirt can get stuck inside easily, and can be very difficult to clean most times. Essential oils such as Patchouli can help reduce oils in the hair by as much as 60% and at the same time stimulate hair regrowth.

Ingredients:

- 2 drops of Patchouli,
- 3 drops of lemongrass oil, and
- 2 drops of Rosemary oil.

Recipe #14: Essential oil treatment for Psoriasis

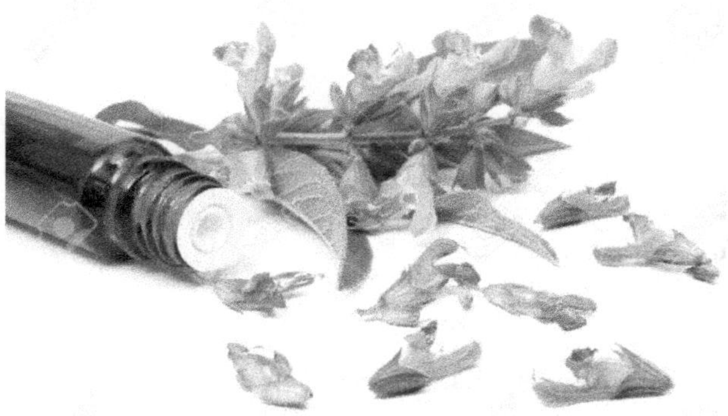

Psoriasis is a hair disorder that can be painful and very difficult to handle. Luckily, essential oils such as Sage and Tea tree can help get rid of this problem gradually because of the powerful antiseptic and antibacterial powers. The essential oils also stimulate healing of the scalp from within. Plants such as Sage can also help clarify the scalp and open it up for the penetration of the healing substances in the oils.

Ingredients:

- 4 drop of oils extracted from Sage plant.
- 3 drops of tea tree oil, and
- 2 drops of rosemary essential oil.

Recipe # 15: The pure and natural skin toner

Are you suffering from pigmentation? Do you age and dark spots you have been trying hard to get rid of? Why not try a blend of Lavender, Palmarosa and Rosewood essential oils. The gentle toning effect of this mix will help you get rid of some skin imperfections within few days. You can spray this essential oil all around your skin through your diffuser, or you can rub it with your hands on your skin.

Ingredients:

- 2 drops of lavender essential oil,
- 8 oz. of distilled water,
- 1 drop of Palmarosa, and
- 1 drop of Rosewood.

Recipe #16: The powerful Body powder

Do you want to feel refreshed and comfortable all day long? Do you want to normalize your skin and get it back to its natural youthful look, even after subjecting yourself to harsh weather conditions? Then this could be the best possible recipe you must consider.

Ingredients:

- 2 tablespoons or 30ml of Corn starch ,
- 10 drops of peppermint essential oil,
- 10 drops of spruce essential oil ,
- 5 drops of Clove essential oil,
- 2 tablespoons of spearmint.

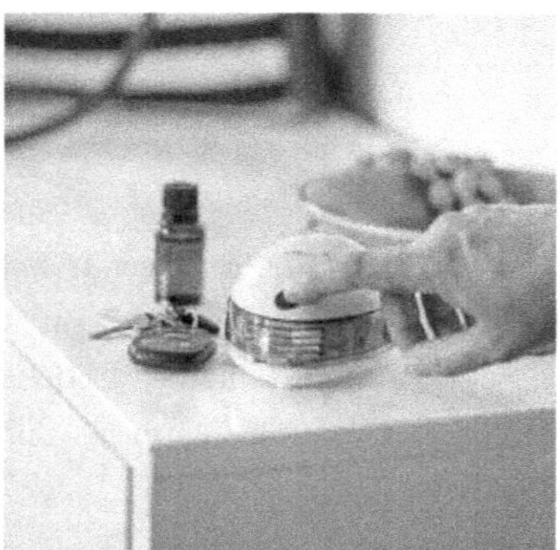

Chapter 4 Diffused essential oil recipes for strengthening immunity/weight loss

Feeling sick quite often, is one of the symptoms of a weakened immunity. Your Immune system may be weakened by a lot of factors, these include; abuse of medications, environmental pollution and poor diets. Here are some essential oil recipes for enhancing immunity;

Recipe #17: The seasonal support recipe

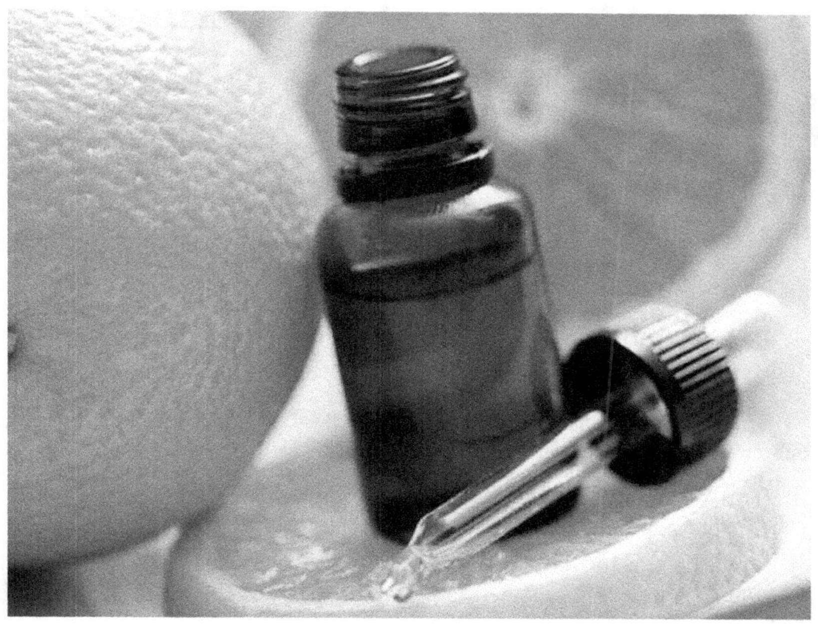

This recipe can help you achieve a clear breathing while strengthening your immunity within a short period of time.

Ingredients:

- 2 drops of peppermint essential oil,
- 1 drop of grape seed essential oil
- 3 drops of lemon oil, and
- 2 drops of orange essential oil

Recipe #18: The fat-buster oils

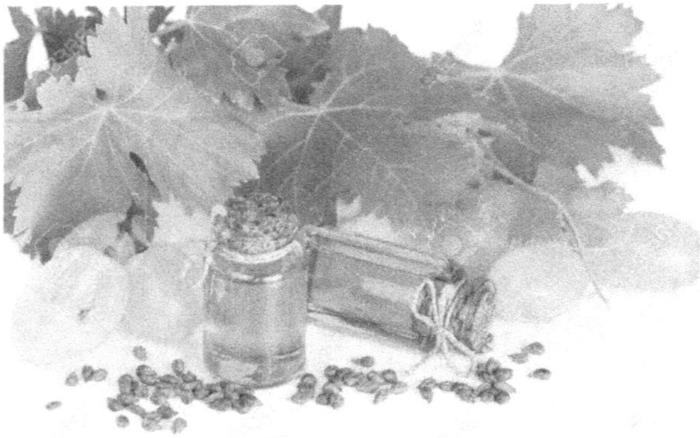

We all know that fruits such as grape fruit and lemon are powerful fat burners. You can mix equal amount of the essential oils of these powerful fruits to obtain their powers. You can also apply the essential oils internally or as a massage. Grapefruit is capable of suppressing appetite , in addition to dissolving fat and increasing energy. Lemon will improve your digestive health, thus speeding up your metabolic rates.

Ingredients:

- 2 drops of Grape seed oil,
- 2 drops of oil extracted from lemon skin.

Recipe #19: appetite suppressant oils

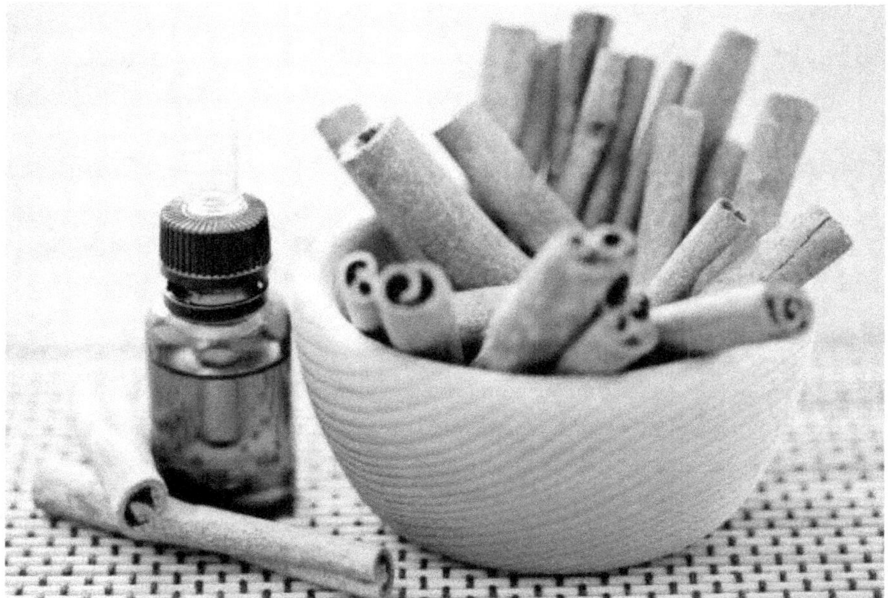

One of the perfect ways of losing weight is to suppress your cravings for food, and there are lots of essential oils that can achieve this. Cinnamon essential oil for instance is capable of boosting your metabolism and at the same time suppress your appetite. Cinnamon is capable of breaking down sugars into energy fast, before they are stored as fat. Peppermint oil can improve digestive health, in addition to providing a soothing effect especially for stomach upset. Peppermint can also make you seem fuller after a moderate meal, therefore you will consume less than you used to.

Ingredients:

- 2 teaspoons of Cinnamon oil
- 2 teaspoons of Peppermint oil.

Recipe #20: The Bergamot oil effect

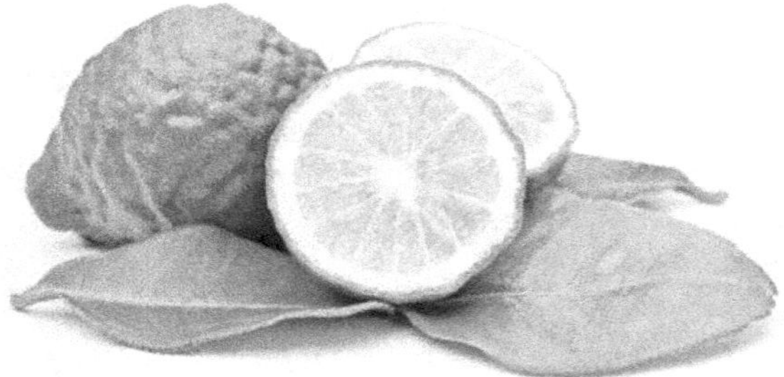

Do you want to inhale the aromatic power of Bergamot and avoid irrational eating? Why not try out Bergamot oil extracts? Bergamot will help you prevent bloating or gassing when you eat excessively. It also helps suppress your appetite or hunger cravings.

Ingredients:

6-8 drops of Bergamot oil extracts.

Recipe # 21: The fat-grounder recipe

This recipe is referred to as the "fat-grounder", because it is capable of creating a net-calorie effect. The recipes here are capable of reducing the amount of fat your body absorbs from each meal; therefore, little or no fat or carb will be stored in in your muscles and body tissues. This effect will eventually help you lose weight at the long run.

Ingredients:

- 2 tablespoons of grapeseed oil,
- 2 tablespoons of lemon oil,
- 2 drops of Vetiver essential oil.

Recipe # 22: The energizing fat burner recipe

FRANKINCENSE OIL:

Used for the Health Benefits for Skin, Arthritis, Age Spots, Women Problems, Blockages

Burning fat should not be the only reason for you to lose weight, you need to maintain a healthy energy level. Fat burning may bring some side effects; include fatigue, slight headache, and loss of sleep. With energizing essential oils such as wild orange and Frankincense, you will definitely rev up your energy levels instantly.

Ingredients:

- 10 drops of Peppermint oil,
- 4 drops of frankincense essential oil,
- 4 drops of Cinnamon essential oil.

Recipe #: The Candy-smell fat buster for kids

Kids will always love the candy smell, and it can be the perfect way to help them lose weight from their young tender age. This recipe can get your kid in shape and you can have some of it too, if you love the smell of candy.

Ingredients:

- 2 drops of wildgreen essential oil,
- 3 drops of wild orange essential oil,
- 1 drop of lime essential oil.

Recipe #23: Goodbye stress, weight loss recipe

Have you ever wonder how the combination of Frankincense, Bergamot and Grapefruit oils will look like? This recipe is not just referred to as stress reliever for nothing; it gives you the perfect mind rest you desire, while you shed that extra weight.

Ingredients:

- 4 drops of Frankincense essential oil,
- 4 drops of Bergamot essential oils,
- 2 drops of Grapeseed essential oil.

Recipe #24: Pathogen killing recipe

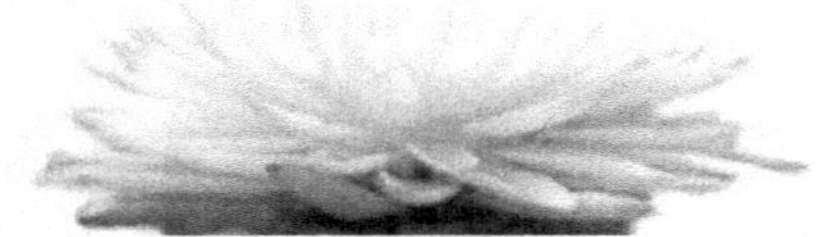

Aside the fact that some weightloss essential oils can burn fat, they also help you get rid of unwanted pathogens in the gut. Lemon and Helichrysum essential oils have been found to be very active in the small and large intestines, thus they can eliminate bacteria, and fungal pathogens quickly before they cause further damages.

Ingredients:

- 4 oz. of distilled water,
- 3 drops of lemon essential oil,
- 1 drop of Helichrysum essential oil.

Recipe #25: system stimulating essential oils

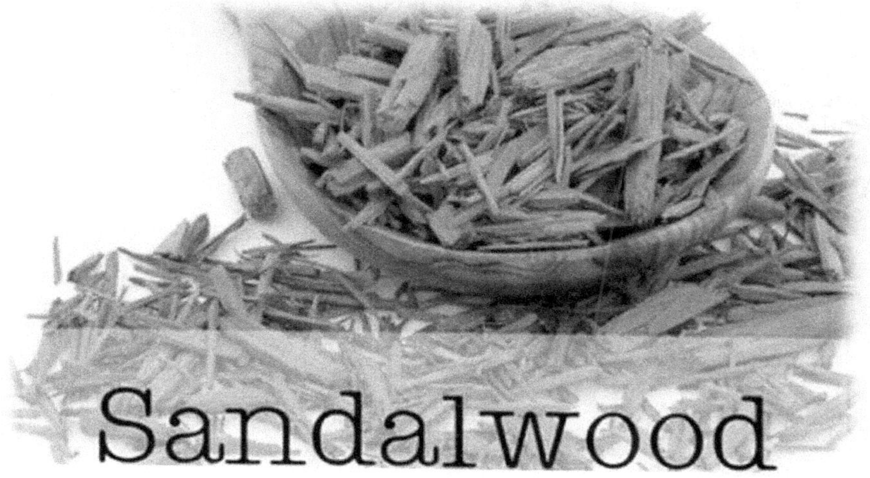

Weight loss don't just happen, there has to be some stimulation effect taking place within the system. For instance, Ginger root oil can help resolve digestive issues that slow down or hinder your weight loss, while

Bergamot essential oil helps fight depression- a psychological disorder that can force you to eat unhealthy food and gain weight quickly. Other essential oils extracted from lime and lemon can help stimulate your nervous system and nourish your body with vitamin C to fight the growth of cellulite. One great thing about this recipe is that it can be applied internally or externally, but make sure the dose for internal application is small, and that can be increased gradually.

Ingredients:

- 2 drops of Ginger root essential oil,
- 2 drops of lime essential oil ,
- 2 drops of Bergamot essential oil, and
- 1 drop of Sandalwood essential oil.

Recipe #26: The anti-cellulite oil blend

If you are overweight, you definitely know how unsightly cellulite will look on your skin, but with the perfect blend of Juniper berry and cypress oil, you can reduce your body's water retention and that means you can get slimmer and smarter always.

Aside taking the oil blend through the mouth, you can consider add some drops of the oil as bath bubbles before transferring it into your bath tub. You need to understand that some essential oils may evaporate quickly; therefore you should add them shortly before you enter the bath.

Ingredients

- 5 drops of Juniper berry essential oil,
- 5 drops of Cypress essential oil,
- 5 drops of orange essential oil (oil extracted from the pulp and skin of orange fruits).

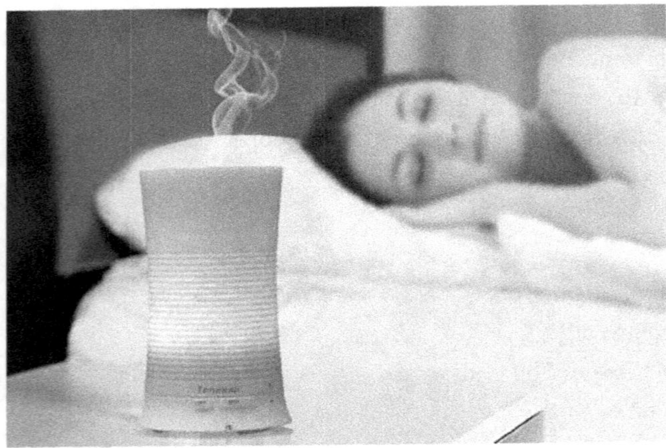

Chapter 5 Diffused essential oil recipes for general health

Bright eyes, balanced blood pressure, mental alertness, and general wellbeing are the ultimate things, every human desire, and fortunately, there are numerous essential oil recipes that can help in achieving these;

Recipe #27: The perfect wind-down essential oil recipe:

Ingredients:

- 4 drops of lavender,
- 2 drops of Cedar wood,
- 2 drops of orange,
- 3 drops of clary sage and
- 1 drop of Marjoram.

Recipe #28: The happy day essential oil recipe

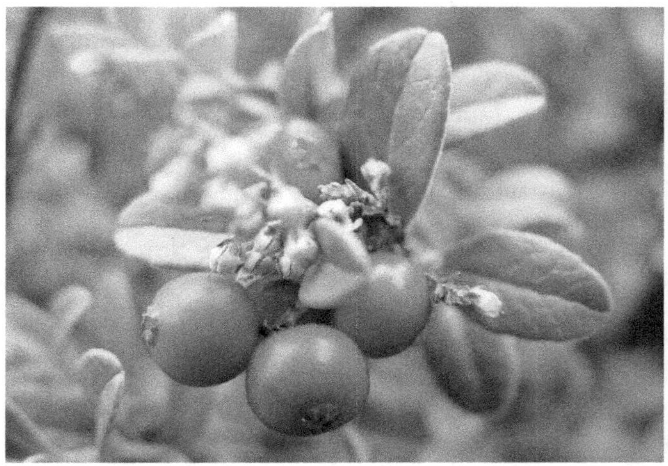

It's the holiday season and you are afraid your kids may have little control over what they put in their mouth. You don't have to stress over this as you can actually help them inhale some natural body cleansers such as white-green and white fir.

Ingredients:

- 1 drop of wintergreen oil,
- 2 drops of white fir, and
- 2 drops of wild orange

Recipe #29: Memory booster/cognitive performance essential oil recipe

Scientists have linked the sniffing of aromatherapy components of plants such as the Spanish sage, to enhance cognitive performance. Spanish sage is believed to contain enzymes that can fight damages to brain cells, thus it can be a vital ingredient in the fight against memory loss and some brain-related problems such as Alzheimer's disease

Ingredients:

- 4 drops of Sage essential oil,
- 2 drops of peppermint oil essential oil.

Recipe#30: The anti-inflammatory and sinus essential oil blends

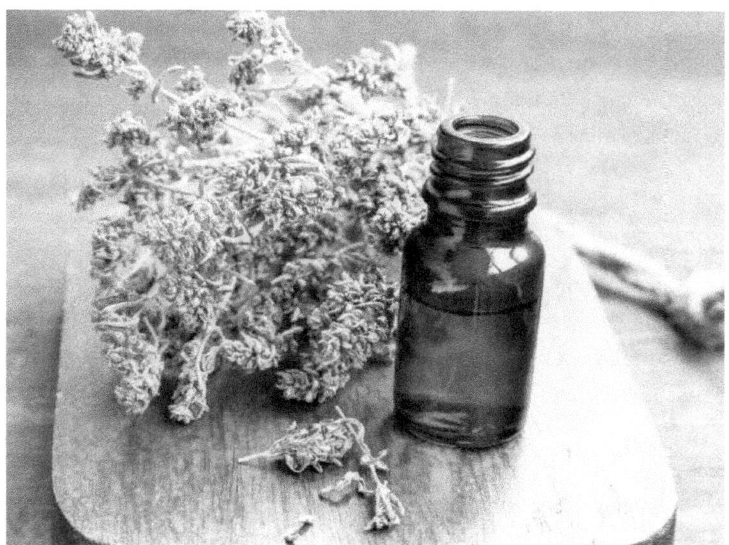

Congestion and headache are often the first symptoms of sinus congestion, this will further become even more unpleasant when cold and allergic reactions cause the blockage of your sinuses and force them to become inflamed. One of the best possible ways of fighting inflammation and other sinus problem is through the use of essential oils such as Eucalyptus, Oregano, menthol, sweet basil, Pine and Thyme.

Ingredients

- 2 drops of Eucalyptus essential oil,
- 2 drops of Oregano essential oil,
- 2 drops of menthol essential oil,
- 2 drops of sweet basil essential oil,
- 2 drops of pine essential oil, and
- 1 drop of thyme essential oil.

Recipe #31: The essential oil blend for allergies

Allergies can arise from many ways, you may develop and allergy from exposure to dirty air, drinking contaminated water, or eating contaminated food. A fine blend of essential oils such as Lemon, Roman Chamomile, Eucalyptus, peppermint, and Lavender, can help alleviate symptoms of allergies.

Ingredients

- 2-3 drops of Lemon,
- 2-4 drops of Roman Chamomile,
- 3 drops of Eucalyptus,
- 2 drops of Peppermint, and
- 2 drops of Lavender.

Recipe #32: Essential oil blend for Migraines and headaches

Headaches and Migraines have become parts of the daily living of most people, instead of spending money on pain and migraine relievers, why not create a fine blend of essential oils such as; Neroli, Jasmine, Balsam fir, Sandalwood, Clove, Valerian, and Helichrysum, that are known to speed up the flow of blood to the brain and give you the much needed freedom from the nagging aches. You don't have to get all these ingredients to prepare your anti-migraine essential oils.

Ingredients:

- 1-2 drops of Neroli essential oil,
- 1-2 drops of Jasmine essential oil,
- 1 drop of Balsam fir,
- 2 drops of Sandalwood,
- 1-2 drops of Clove
- 2 drops of Valerian, and
- 1 drop of Helichrysum.

Recipe #33: The Face blend for sensitive skin

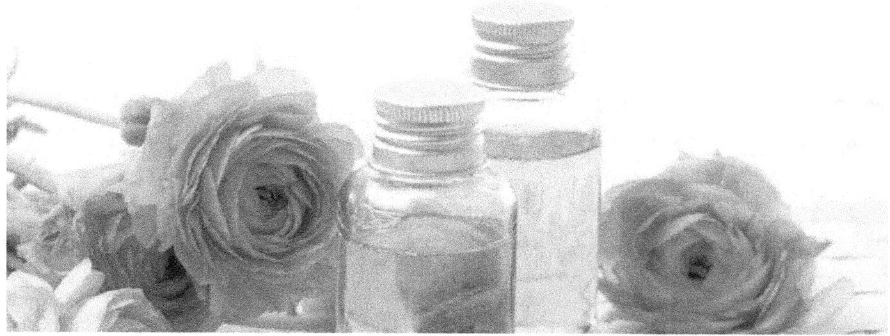

This could be the ideal blend for individuals suffering from over-sensitive skin, especially when the skin turns red or develop any form of allergic reaction to extreme heat , sunlight or extra bright light. The addition of almond oil in this recipe can serve as a moisturizing oil.

Ingredients

- 2 drops of Frankincense oil,
- 1 drop of Rose oil,
- A tablespoon of sweet almond oil.

Recipe #34: anti corn and calluses essential oils

Corns and calluses often appear on the feet and their sight can be unsightly, especially when you are enjoying outdoor activities, with lots of people. If you want to return your feet to normal before the summer season, then this should be the right time to act.

Ingredient:

- 2 tablespoons of sweet almond oil (sun flower oil can also be used in place of this),
- 12 drops of lavender essential oil, and
- 10 drops of carrot seed oil.

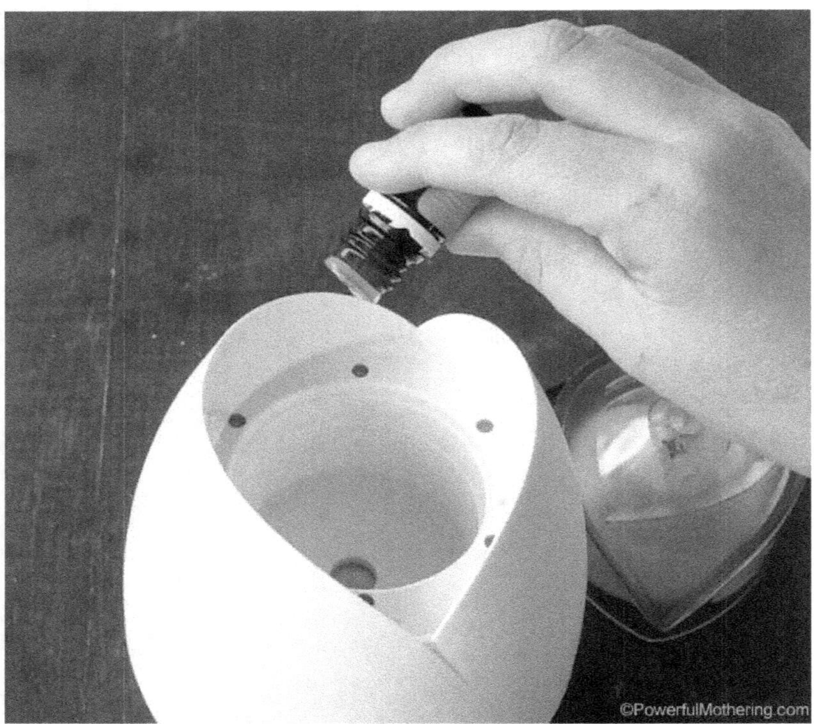

Chapter 6 Diffused essential oil recipes for clean environment

An inviting environment is very important, and fortunately there are lots of diffused essential oil recipes that can take care of this aspect effectively.

Recipe #35: The Fresh and clean essential oil recipes

Ingredients

- 1-2 drops of lavender oil,
- 2 drops of lemon essential oil, and
- 2 drops of Rosemary essential oil.

This essential oil should last for several days when used once or twice a day from inside the diffuser.

Recipe # 36: The Odour eliminator essential

If you have lots of pets or kids that get messy often, you need to fresh the air with some de-odourants. This recipe is surely a perfect one any day.

Ingredients:

- 2 drops of Malaleuca essential oil,
- 2 drops of lemon oil,
- 1 drop of lime essential oil, and
- 1 drop of Cilantro oil.

Recipe #37: The insect repellant recipe

You don't have to waste your money on dangerous chemical repellants for cockroaches, flies and other crawling and flying insects. Simply follow this recipe;

Ingredient:

- 1 drop of lemon grass,
- 1 drop of tea tree,
- 1 drop of Thyme,
- 1 drop of Eucalyptus.

Recipe #38: the extra-clean essential oil recipe

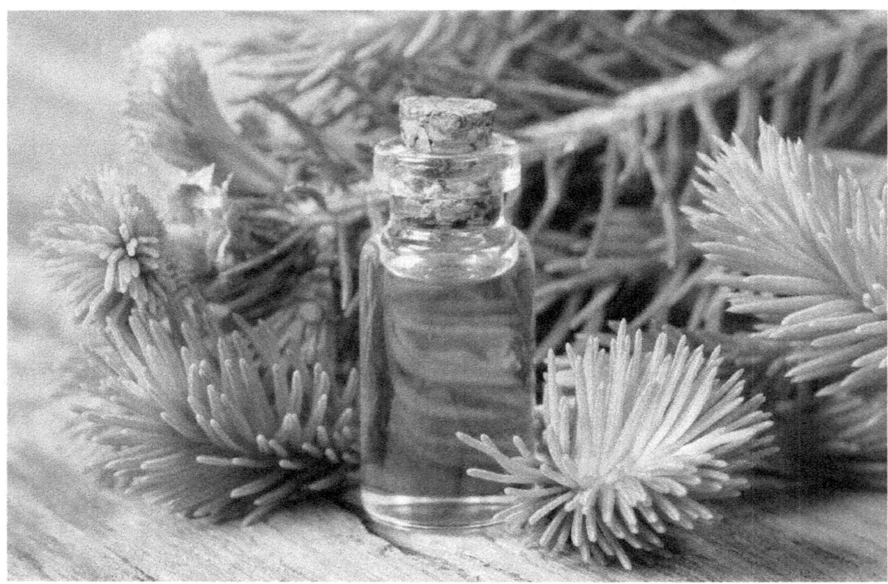

Sometimes, you just have to do more than cleaning the surface, you need essential oils that clean and sanitize to ensure a perfect sterile environment.

Essential oils extracted from Pine, for instance, are capable of destroying pathogenic spores, therefore, such oils can be used in getting rid of molds in the bathroom, and can also be used to clean the floor where they can leave natural scents.

Ingredients:

- 5 drops of essential oils of Pine,
- 5 drops of essential oils from Cinnamon leaf, and
- 5 drops of essential oils extracted from Thyme.

Recipe #39: The most re-invigourating essential oils for the interior

When it comes to re-invigourating the interior of your home, three top cleaning essential oils come to mind and these are; Lavender, Eucalyptus and Peppermint. Peppermint is always cool around the home and this is why it is found in spray cleaners, and natural deodourants.

Eucalyptus is an excellent germicide that can be used in dry-washing the dirtiest stuffs around, while Vinegar and lavender can be paired together to give some soothing scent and this is why they are found in many products, including linen sprays, and dish soap.

Ingredients:

- 3 drops of lavender essential oil, mixed with a drop of Vinegar,
- 2 drops of Eucalyptus essential oil, and
- 2 drops of peppermint oil.

Recipe #40: The perfect degreasing essential oil recipe for the most stubborn stains

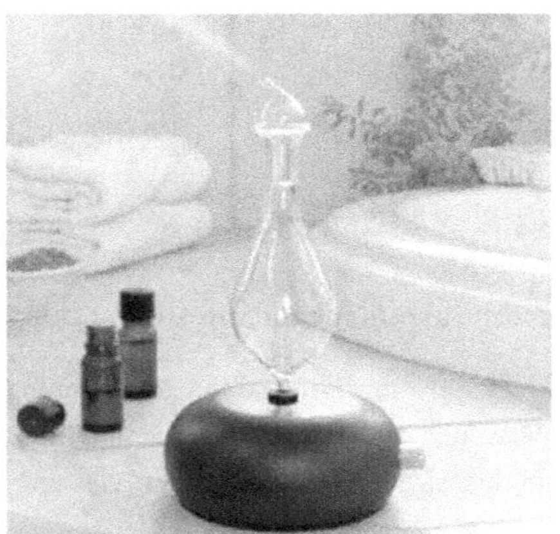

You don't have to spend your hard earned money on bleach or degreasing chemicals when you can make use of common homemade essential oils like Melaleuca (tea tree), rosemary, lemon and wild orange. Tea tree can be the best handy potent weapon against bugs, while lemon can be used to freshen up items such as the refrigerator because they can stick to the stubborn stains. Rosemary is found in Laundry detergents and soaps because it is a natural antiseptic.

Ingredients:

- 4 drops of lavender essential oil,
- 3 drops of tea tree oil essential oil,
- 4 drops of rosemary essential oil, and,
- 3 drops of lemon essential oils.

Conclusion

In order to get the best out of your essential oil mix, you need to ensure that your diffuser is perfectly screwed or capped, to ensure that there are no leakages or exposure of the components of the oils.

When essential oils are exposed to gas, and light, they tend to lose their strength and that means they may not perform at their optimal levels. You need to ensure that you store your essential oils under room conditions, whether they are inside the diffuser or not. If possible, place them inside an enclosure and far away from where their volatile constituents can be adequately covered.

It is also important that you stick with the doses of each essential oil as the overdose of some essential oils has been found to cause certain side effects. Whether they are inhaled or ingested through the mouth. You need to have a check on your body's ability to withstand even the small doses recommended in this book.

This book has provided the minimal safe dose for each addition of the essential oil within a mix; therefore it is important that you stick with them. Essential oil should be started with low doses and can be increased steadily as your body can tolerate them.

Hope you enjoy deriving the utmost results from all essential oils mentioned in this book.

FREE Bonus Reminder

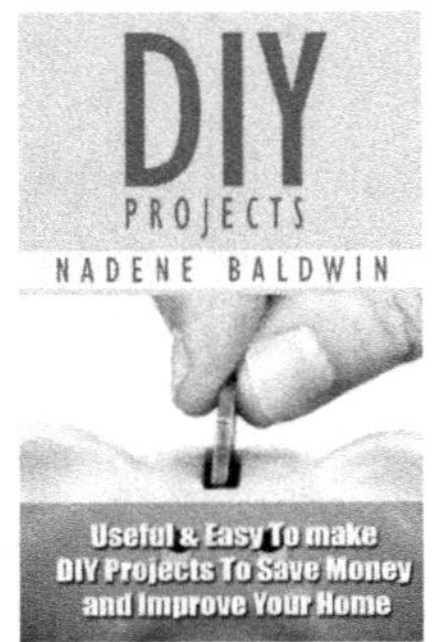

If you have not grabbed it yet, please go ahead and download your special bonus report *"DIY Projects. 13 Useful & Easy To Make DIY Projects To Save Money & Improve Your Home!"*

Simply Click the Button Below

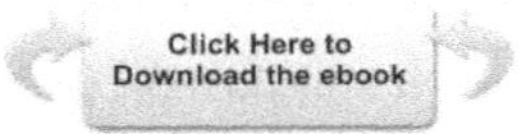

OR **Go to This Page**

http://diyhomecraft.com/free

BONUS #2: More Free & Discounted Books

Do you want to receive more Free & Discounted Books?

We have a mailing list where we send out our new Books when they go free or with a discount on Kindle. Click on the link below to sign up for Free & Discount Book Promotions.

=> Sign Up for Free & Discount Book Promotions <=

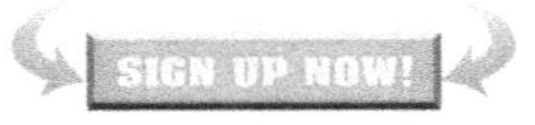

OR Go to this URL

http://zbit.ly/1WBb1Ek

www.ingramcontent.com/pod-product-compliance
Lightning Source LLC
Chambersburg PA
CBHW060819260726
48660CB00003B/1006